I0788077

# HOW TO DEFINITIVELY CURE CHRONIC INSOMNIA

STOP BEING AWAKE AT 3 AM IN THE MORNING, ELIMINATE NOCTURNAL WAKEFULNESS, ANXIETY AND NERVES WITH NATURAL TREATMENTS

Jorge O. Chiesa

Copyright 2019© Jorge O. Chiesa

All rights reserved. No part of this publication may be reproduced or distributed in any form or by any means, electronic or mechanical, including photocopying, recording, or by any information storage or retrieval system, without the prior written permission of the authors.

First Edition

# Table of Contents

## *Introduction The Science Behind Insomnia*

Have you ever suffered from insomnia? In other words, do you face the difficulty of falling asleep and staying asleep at night? So what causes it?

Insomnia is often caused by multiple reasons, such as not getting enough rest, hunger, psychological trauma, etc. No matter what the reason, millions of human beings suffer from the devil called insomnia. It prevents you from getting enough rest, depletes your energy and destroys your productivity the next day. Not to mention the detrimental effect on their own physical and mental health.

## *What is insomnia?*

Insomnia by definition is the difficulty of falling asleep and staying asleep. This refers to the types of restlessness that a person suffers at different points in their sleep cycle. A simple

The indication for diagnosing insomnia is when a person is not satisfied with the amount of sleep they have been sleeping.

Those with insomnia:

They will feel a lack of energy, fatigue at different times of the day, having difficulty concentrating on tasks, experiencing terrible mood swings, and having a low level of performance in the workplace.

Insomniacs may have any of these conditions


Symptoms after staying up all night:


A human body requires rest to rejuvenate both mind and body. The lack of rest in any of them will cause fatigue and various mental illnesses. Although they are terribly exhausted to the core, they still cannot fall asleep or do not fall asleep due to different causes.

# *The two types of insomnia*

## 1.  *Acute Insomnia*

There are two main types of insomnia. The first type is the type of insomnia when you only have a couple of restless nights. Often, you can fall asleep and stay asleep easily. For many, insomniacs may not think they are suffering from it, but the fact is that they may be having acute insomnia.

So, what is acute insomnia? This type of insomnia comes from the basic levels of stress that insomniacs are experiencing at that time. They will face a short period of time in which they will not be able to fall asleep due to the life circumstances they face at that time. This kind of insomnia doesn't last long. Instead, it only occurs due to certain factors or events during a specific time period.

For example, acute insomnia can occur after insomniacs face their boss's anger, get a poor grade on an exam, are rejected for falling in love, or simply because they are having a "bad day. These situations can cause a person to have one or two nights when they simply can't sleep. Many people may have experienced this type of insomnia and it tends to resolve itself.

## 2.  *Chronic Insomnia*

The second type of insomnia is known as chronic insomnia. Insomnia is a type of prolonged insomnia that occurs at least three nights a week and lasts for at least three months. This usually occurs when you are faced with a significant change in your environment, physically or mentally. It can be moving to a new home, losing a loved one, being in a new workplace, facing challenges at school, or having trouble adapting to a more severe climate. Perhaps the reason chronic insomniacs are having trouble sleeping is because they have an unhealthy sleep habit without a proper sleep routine.

It is common in today's world; modern society has ruined the sleep cycle with short hours of sleep. To make matters worse, most of them sleep at strange hours. They don't practice the habit of going to bed early and getting up early the next day.

As a result, the mind doesn't know when to close and would be used to staying up late. That is why insomnia has become a common problem in today's society. What people don't understand is that the body won't be able to function with a small amount of sleep one night and hopes to make up for their lack of sleep by taking naps later in the day. While this may seem possible and useful at first, this sleep pattern is not sustainable in the long term.

Eventually, the mind and body will collapse, and you will experience total exhaustion until you get enough rest. The best solution is to have a fixed sleep schedule and practice a healthy sleep routine. Otherwise, you need to visit your doctor to get medicine. It will typically be related to another medical or psychiatric problem, which means that the reason you may be having chronic insomnia is due to stress. What appears to be a typical situation will seem stressful if you have chronic insomnia. A restless mind and body will be bothered by any stimulus from the immediate environment.

## *The causes of insomnia*

Regardless of the types of insomnia, the causes are the following

the same thing. The difference lies in the intensity of the emotions that a person experiences during a given time.

In addition to that, underlying medical conditions can also cause insomnia. Fortunately, insomnia is treatable in most cases.

These medical conditions may be severe or mild, inducing insomnia to occur at a different time in a person's life. These symptoms include nasal allergies, sinus allergies, low back pain, chronic general pain, gastrointestinal problems, arthritis, asthma, and other neurological problems.

The stress on the patient's body will cause the mind to remain awake for a longer period of time. For example, those who catch a cold will find that they stay awake most of the night or that they wake up frequently. Both factors can result in a person with a severe lack of sleep and rest. They may try to relax while they have a cold, but insomnia will prevail.

Physical pain can also cause insomnia because the body cannot put itself in a comfortable position to rest. Have you ever experienced sleepless nights because you cannot put yourself in a comfortable position? This situation is typical when you experience any pain in your body. The best way to fall asleep and stay asleep quickly is to put your body in a comfortable position in bed. It will also help in healing and ensure a more productive sleep. Otherwise, you'll find yourself in a constant battle to fall asleep and even opt for unnecessary medications if you can't adopt your best sleeping posture.

With all these different causes in mind, we can now move on to the cure. But it is equally important to study all the factors that

Cause insomnia. But did you know that there are also risk factors for insomnia? If you find that some of these risks apply to you, then you simply have a greater chance of having insomnia at some point in your life. Otherwise, pay attention to your health and sleep habits to make sure you are insomnia-free for the rest of your life.

# *Risk factors for insomnia*

Risk factors for insomnia include being a woman, being pregnant or in the menopause period, adults over the age of forty, suffering from more stress, suffering from depression, having a night job, traveling long distances where there is a time change, or having a family history of insomnia. All of these factors bring a person closer to insomnia. But do you realize that most of these risk factors are the result of your choices? In most cases, people think they have little or no choice in life, which is not true.

They may choose to take a longer vacation when they move through different time zones, but they did not. They may look for a day job, but they decided to go through the difficult times of having a night job and adapting to a completely different lifestyle.

It is difficult to deal with the risk factors of insomnia, but ultimately it all depends on your choices. Sometimes, you can have a hard time in life. They can be problems of couple, family or work. Not only that, you could be suffering from financial or personal problems where you are having trouble balancing your professional and personal life. All of this will hit you and keep you awake at night until most of the stress or depression is gone. In some cases, it may take longer. In other cases, people can find solutions and overcome difficult times fairly quickly. Either way, having the right mentality is the cure for emotion-induced insomnia.

Because insomnia has many different causes and risk factors, there are many different things you can do to keep you from having more sleepless nights and restlessness. Most of the time, it's easy to find out what the causes are, but the real challenge is how to get over it and have a good night's sleep. Life can be difficult, and sometimes it can hit a person to the point where they're not even sure if they can get up again.

The first step in overcoming insomnia is not to be afraid. Don't be afraid of any outcome that may or may not happen. Fear produces more stress in your life than it serves you. In fact, he can only intensify his insomnia. Prevention is always better than cure. Always remember to stay calm and follow health tips to avoid insomnia.

## *The mind of a person with insomnia*

Researchers around the world are joining their minds to find out how an insomniac's brain works. They continue to look at the characteristics of all brain waves and how thoughts interact during the day and night.

### ➢ *How the mind works*

During each hour of the day, the mind is able to adapt to any new situation. Whether you're trying to get food, have a drink, get out of the car, walk through a door or just rest a bit, the mind will constantly try to find new ways to survive and thrive. You will continue through the cycle of getting enough resources during the day and will have enough energy to heal and rest during the night.

Normally, people with a healthy level of brain waves with satisfactory cognitive stability during the day are able to turn off parts of the brain waves.

> ***Brain thinking***

During the night. As the night falls deeper, the brain will begin to slow down and start sleeping. Their alertness and concentration typically decrease at night. This is why one person finds it more difficult to complete any task at night.

Studies show that the process of the mind will naturally change throughout the day, and sometimes cause a greater form of anxiety. It is when brain waves become erratic and refuse to slow down due to an immense amount of stress during the day. Therefore, the mind will not be able to relax completely at night. Instead, you will go through a period when brain waves will move unusually fast, causing more thoughts and consuming more energy at night. Everything a person has gone through during the day will be picked up at night. The body will then go through twice as much energy and resources to process the thoughts, and this causes fatigue and lack of energy the next day.

> ### ➢ *The mind and brain waves*

As for the mind and how brain waves respond to the phases of insomnia, there are three different studies to show how the brain reacts during the night. Brain learning and memory processing functions have been shown to affect a person's sleep. The more you learn during the day, the more thoughts and memories will be processed by the brain during the night.

Dreams come from one's own real life thoughts and experiences. The more you experience in life, the more you dream at night. The ability to have a greater variety of dreams allows the mind to calm down and form vague images to reinforce its memory. When you fall into a deep sleep, you tend to be in the dream state. Sometimes you can even have nightmares. But everything boils, even your subconscious thoughts and the kind of experience you had.

## *Day vs. Night*

What's going on in the insomniac brain? First, your brain is more active during the night and has difficulty reaching a state of calm and relaxation. In one of the studies on brain waves during insomnia, scientists have shown that the neurons of the insomniac's brain are most active during the night.

Insomniacs tend to have many thoughts going through their heads, resulting in insomnia. They are experiencing a constant state of information processing throughout the day without the ability to stop it. Ultimately, they will have insomnia and face the consequences of not having enough rest.

Experts say insomnia should not be seen directly as a nighttime disorder. In fact, it's more of a 24-hour brain condition that keeps the brain active all day long.

Sleep plays an important role in the processing and storage of memories. Lack of sleep will interfere with your long-term memory. You will have trouble concentrating, remembering facts and even minor details. This theory was tested with a group of students in a short test. One group slept all night, while another group did not sleep the night before. The results? Students who slept more could concentrate more, and could remember their answers to the test a few hours later. The group of students who didn't get enough sleep struggled with the test, scored below average, and barely remember the answers they wrote an hour after the test.

## *The Myths*

The aim of this experiment is to demonstrate the importance of rest for a person's focus and memory. In fact, insomniacs can't have the same level of concentration as those who rested enough. Surprisingly, some people believe they may have the same attention span during the day. The fact that the brain is as active at night as it is during the day does not mean that the brain can function at its maximum level.

In addition to lack of concentration, research shows that Insomnia has more brain plasticity. However, research on what plasticity is and how it contributes to states of insomnia is still unknown. But what they do know is that brain plasticity accumulates throughout a person's life and contributes to other forms of disease later on. Brain plasticity is the brain's ability to change structurally and functionally in response to physical or environmental factors.

In most cases, brain plasticity allows us to absorb new information, learn new things, and continue to grow over time.

Adulthood. But in the case of insomnia, it damages brain cells and leads to brain plasticity. This leads to poor memory retention and lack of concentration. Not only in the short term, but also in the long term. It's harder to hold on to all levels of concentration and memory as a person ages.

# The brain of the restless mind

Other research was done to find out how stress and anxiety affect sleep. The goal was to determine if a person with a stressful lifestyle has insomnia and how the brain responds at night. And here's the result: The cognitive function of the brain doesn't change whether they have insomnia or not. However, insomniacs find it more difficult to concentrate and process information throughout the day.

Most research shows that the mind of insomniacs wanders during the night. They will have difficulty concentrating the next day; they will face challenges in managing their work, their studies and even their personal lives.

In other words, the mind will have difficulty functioning optimally the next day and insomniacs will not be able to perform at their best. Another part of the research compared memory, function, and efficiency to complete any task given to insomniacs and those who had enough rest.

Studies show that insomniacs are unable to remember most of their memories during the day. As a result, they face difficulties in completing their daily tasks. Their minds would wander even when they are performing simple tasks. For example, when it comes to preparing breakfast, people with a healthy amount of sleep will go to the kitchen, make quick decisions and start their day. On the other hand, those who suffer from insomnia will enter the kitchen, end up opening more cabinets, looking through the same food, and unable to figure out what they should have for breakfast.

**_And here's the explanation_**: An insomniac's brain waves are slower, and this will cause him or her to move at a slower pace and forget simple things quickly. In addition, as they progress through the day and more tasks are presented, the prefrontal cortex will begin to have fewer resources, and brain waves will become erratic. The brain will try to stay active, but it won't have enough energy to process everything. Therefore, the brain will eventually run out if you are suffering from insomnia.

## *Gray Matter*

The third and final scientific study is to determine the role of brain gray matter. The most important thing to know about gray matter is that it exists in the frontal lobe and controls the processes of memory and executive function. When insomniacs do not get enough sleep at night, they will have a substantial decrease in gray matter. Whether they are suffering from insomnia or having trouble sleeping in general, they will begin to develop symptoms of depression or trauma slowly. The underlying cause of insomnia is usually stress. The best way to solve this problem is to consult a doctor to find out which type of medicine would be best for you.

In short, the mind has to get enough

sleep and rest to have adequate concentration. Insomnia will only put your body into overdrive mode and therefore you will not be resting enough. The next important thing to remember is to get enough nutrition and sleep every night. No matter how difficult it is to find a balance, it is important to have a high level of concentration every day to get the most out of your day.

## *The most negative thing about insomnia*

In the last chapter, the mind was explored to understand how insomnia directly affects the brain. Having this disorder for any amount of time will cause a massive negative impact on the mind. In addition to memory loss, insomnia also causes tiredness, carelessness, and lack of alertness the next day. Mind and body need rest to function well the next day. If there is no rest, then gray matter, memory, and the elaborate duties of the mind will crumble, and insomniacs will have difficulty passing the day. Your mind will wander, and you will struggle to stay focused throughout the day.

## *The 5 things you do every morning*

Here's a little exercise: First, try to think of all the things you did the moment you wake up today. Reflect on the first five things you did. You can turn off the alarm clock, check the phone, stand up, turn on the lights and walk to the bathroom. No matter what your usual routine is, you tend to execute all your regular activities impeccably. Believe it or not, you subconsciously perform all these activities without thinking much, just because it became a daily routine.

However, when you have insomnia, you are not as focused as you normally are. The mind will continue to think as fast as it normally would, but it does not have all the resources and energy to function properly. In short, you may find it difficult to do your first five activities in the morning, and you may have difficulty completing each task.

An easy way to know this is when you realize that it took you longer than it should have to perform these tasks. The five actions that are supposed to take only 2 minutes to complete can end up taking more than 10 minutes when you haven't rested enough. You may even forget to do one or two tasks. You may forget to turn off the alarm and forget to check your phone for updates. Many different things can happen, but in general this is only the tip of the iceberg when you are struggling with insomnia.

# *Damaging your professional life*

After the first night you face insomnia, you may notice a significant decrease in your energy level. You may find it difficult to plan the day, or you may find it harder to remember all the information during the day.

In most cases, your daily routine can begin with waking up, preparing for work, or even shopping afterwards. All jobs require a 100% approach to ensure high performance and efficiency. Otherwise, you may have to face your boss's music. No matter how exhausted you feel, there are only a certain number of days when you will be given sympathy. There is a limited number of sick leaves you can take in a year. So don't let insomnia destroy your personal and professional life. Take charge and get rid of him once and for all.

   At your job, you are expected to complete tasks by a certain deadline. Whether you're in charge of packing boxes, doing research or writing, you have to be at the top of your game almost every day. You have to perform at peak all the time and earn your well-deserved paycheck at the end of the month. Any rest sacrificed during the night can result in poor performance the next day.

## *Do you experience lack of sleep?*

Each person has his or her own sleep rhythm, and experts recommend 6 to 8 hours of sleep each day. The exact number depends on the individual. Some of us need more rest, some less. But at the end of the day, losing a couple of hours of sleep is always better than losing an entire night's rest. For example, instead of getting eight hours of sleep, you only get six hours of sleep. Those two hours of sleep may seem crucial, but they won't do as much damage to your life as insomnia. Losing two hours of sleep can slow you down, but chances are you'll still be able to get ahead and do all the tasks at the end of the day. On the other hand, losing an entire night's sleep can shut down your brain. They will spend the day struggling with simple tasks.

For example, when your boss puts an address book on your desk, you can read the content without problems. But realizing what each item on the list means is the hard part for people with insomnia. What appears to be a walk in the park may seem like an impossible mission for insomniacs.

Often, you lose concentration and the purpose of the day if you don't sleep. You would be constantly looking for the fastest way to spend the day instead of thinking about the best way to spend the day. At first, it may seem manageable because you can still do things on time from time to time. But the truth is that, in the long run, it will damage your reputation in the workplace because of the poor quality of your work. Moreover, insomniacs are known to have a bad temper and a bad working relationship with their colleagues.

People will notice your inefficiency eventually. Your boss will notice that you are working at a slower pace, that you are not concentrating as much, and that you do not have the right attitude to complete the job. You can put him in the wrong favor of your boss, and you could also risk getting fired. Although this may seem unlikely at this time, you should keep in mind that the possibility is very high. Insomnia is a distressing factor in life that can cause problems not only in the workplace, but also in your personal life.

# Damaging your personal life

When you think of your personal life, think of all that is important to you, the things you carry in your heart. You might think of your wife, husband, children, pets or any other aspect. Some people may even think about their garden or the remodeling project they've been working on.

There is no right or wrong answer to this. It's your own life, and the key to success in your personal life is balance. Most people go about their daily routine without thinking much about it. Some examples are simple tasks such as making breakfast for your children, getting in the car, or going somewhere to eat.

Normally, these are not difficult tasks, but insomniacs may feel the opposite. The moment a person's personal life begins to unbalance, this results in stressful moments, and they begin to question whether there is any way to return to a stable state.

Whether the stress comes from not having groceries on time or waking up late, a minimal amount of stress can build up in something out of control. Insomnia causes a significant amount of stress and exhaustion.

There will be no specific thought in your mind; your mind will only wander with random thoughts without context. The same applies to your working life. If you suffer from insomnia and need to prepare your children for school, you may miss your lunch box, forget to iron your clothes and the list goes on.

Always remember to put yourself first as "Self-love is NOT selfish". When you constantly put yourself in last place, you will find yourself in a downward spiral of life, unable to fulfill your ultimate purpose in life.

Now is the time to unveil a great misunderstanding in our society, the perception of putting oneself first as arrogant, evil and selfish. What they didn't understand is that if you are busy fulfilling the demands of others without achieving the purposes of your life, you would feel dissatisfied and doomed. You would lose your drive, motivation, enthusiasm and productivity if you went down this road. So stop pleasing others and prioritize yourself first. Only then will you have an unstoppable drive to achieve more, and you will have more to offer in return.

At home, you may have to keep your home by mowing the lawn or walking around the house to check for insects. No matter what you do, you must remember the steps to execute each action accurately. The moment you suffer from insomnia, you will not be able to remember things very well, and it will be more difficult for you to do so.

Another vital part of your personal life is your relationship with others. Whether your partner, husband, wife, boyfriend or girlfriend, being in a relationship is a job in itself. If you don't pay full attention to your partner because you didn't get enough rest, then you can expect your relationship to crack. This situation will lead to arguments, dissatisfaction, frustration, loneliness and sadness in a relationship. All of these emotions can reach a point where a major confrontation may be necessary.

# Dealing With Insomnia

It's hard to deal with insomnia when there's no energy left inside you. You will feel tired all the time and care less about the things that are happening around you. Your mind will wander, and many times those thoughts make no sense at all. Life itself is hard enough. Now, imagine adding the fact that you're not resting and have to deal with all the obstacles life presents to you. How would you feel? Overwhelmed? Stressed?

You could end up wasting your time at your workplace. You may not prepare meals as a family and may upset your children. You could start forgetting all the little things that normally do for your romantic relationship. Many areas in your life can go south because of insomnia.

With all of this in mind, now is the time to protect yourself from sleep loss and get optimal rest every night.

## The Cure: Natural and Artificial Remedies

Sleep is incredibly important to health. We need to sleep so that our body heals and rejuvenates from the activities of our day. Unfortunately, many people have difficulty falling asleep or simply don't get enough sleep, which is where insomnia remedies come into play.

There are two basic categories when it comes to insomnia remedies.

> ## Artificial Remedy

The first is the Artificial Remedy. This type of medicine can be found in the pharmacy and clinic. They are usually prescribed to treat the disease at its source. Artificial remedies usually cost a pump, but typically give quick results. Most of today's medications are toxic, filled with harmful chemicals that are not safe to be consumed for an extended period of time.

> ***Natural Remedy***

The other type of remedy is called Natural Remedy. People have practiced natural medicine for centuries. This type of remedy uses the body's natural healing process to fight insomnia. It is often less expensive, but what makes them stand out is the fact that they are not as toxic as Artificial Remedies.

Regardless of the type of remedy you choose, the goal is to help you fall asleep and stay asleep. These remedies are meant to help you get more rest at night. Most of these remedies cause drowsiness, so it's best to take them just before bedtime, unless otherwise noted. It is also important to make sure you talk to a doctor before taking any of the medicines listed below.

- Eszopiclone: Also known as Lunesta, is a group of drugs able to put you to sleep easily and quickly. Statistics show that Lunesta is able to put most people to sleep for an average of 7-8 hours. It's a strong drug group, so be sure to stay away from it unless you can get a full night's rest to prevent drowsiness. The FDA limits the dose of the drug to no more than 1 mg. Anything else could cause the risk of stunning the next day.

• Ramelteon: This group of drugs works differently, does not cause adverse effects to users such as dizziness, drowsiness, etc.. The common drugs used to induce sleep are directed to the CNS (Central Nervous System), depressing its functions and putting the user into a sleep state. Ramelteon, on the other hand, focuses specifically on the sleep-wake cycle. This medicine is prescribed for people who have difficulty falling asleep. Due to the lack of side effects, Ramelteon can be prescribed for long-term use. The drug has also shown no history of abuse or dependence.

• Zaleplon: Also known as Sonata. Most drugs have a long activation time in the human body. Sonata is not one of them. Among the latest sleeping pills, Sonata managed to stay active in the system for as short a time as possible. In other words, this medicine leaves few or no side effects the next morning. For example, if a person has difficulty falling asleep, a Sonata tablet will help them fall asleep without feeling bad the next day.

• Doxepin: Also known as Silenor. This group of medications is prescribed specifically for those who have difficulty staying asleep. It can be said that it is an artificial remedy for "light sleepers" who wake up easily at night thanks to a minimum amount of stimuli. It works by suppressing histamine receptors, thus helping to maintain sleep after you have fallen asleep. As this medicine requires you to stay asleep for a certain time, do not take Silenor unless you can sleep up to 7-8 hours a night. The dose depends on your response to treatment, health, and age.

- Benzodiazepines:

Benzodiazepines are useful for both short-term and long-term insomnia. It has a lasting effect on the body, as it remains in the system for a long time. Therefore, for those who have had insomnia for a long time, this medication may help them on their journey toward full recovery.

It is commonly used to treat prolonged nightmares and sleepwalking. Because the effect of this drug is inflexible, you may feel tired and drowsy the next day. Another side effect of this medication is that this medication can result in drug dependence, which means that you may have to rely on this medication to fall asleep and stay asleep in the future.

Benzodiazepines can be found in the sleeping pills Triazolam (Halcion), Alprazolam (Xanax), Temazepam (Restoril), and others.

It is important to have a medical evaluation before taking any sleeping pill. See a doctor for a complete exam. Always

Talk to your doctor about the adverse effects of any medication before deciding which pills to take. Each medicine can cause different side effects. Side effects may include headache, severe allergic reactions, prolonged drowsiness, to name just a few.

On the other hand, some would prefer natural remedies. You don't have to rely on chemicals with harmful adverse effects, especially on waking. Instead, why not use natural remedies to repair your sleep cycle and put an end to insomnia?

## *Camping*

When the attraction of television or touching the phone keeps you awake late into the night, it's time to pick up the tent and go camping. Stay away from electronic devices and enjoy digital detox from time to time. Put yourself in a distraction-free zone and be aware of your environment and yourself. Use this time to meditate, do some yoga, write, remember your thoughts or just breathe.

According to several studies, campers who stay away from appliances and practice rituals such as meditating or listening to music fall asleep about 2 hours earlier than usual. Another important point to remember is that digital devices contribute to insomnia. Artificial light sources have been found to adversely affect circadian rhythms.

Try sleeping on the floor, not in the car or in the cockpit. That way, you'll be punished and you'll be one with nature. Regardless of what you do during camp, the ultimate goal is to relax, to get away from the distractions and demands of others, to get away from artificial light and to be one with nature. Bathe in natural sunlight and fall asleep when the sun sets. In the blink of an eye, you'll restore your sleep rhythms.

## *Music Therapy*

Music has been used since ancient times to combat insomnia. It is a healing tool that can help alleviate anxiety that can contribute to poor sleep quality. The biggest advantage of this technique is that it is easy to use and has no side effects.

There are many different types of music therapy and they differ in the types of neurological stimulation they evoke. For example, classical music can be a powerful tool for comfort and relaxation, while rock music can cause discomfort. Try to go for soft and relaxing music that has nature sounds like the ocean, birds, waterfalls, etc.

Several studies showed that people who

listen to soothing music before bedtime improved the quality of sleep during the night than people who don't listen to it. Therefore, if you have trouble falling asleep, this may be a solution.

# *Off for a better rest*

Sleep is not an on/off switch. Your body needs time to relax and prepare for sleep. Insomniacs often have trouble shutting down their brains at night. You can try turning off the equipment to get a better night's sleep. This technique helps calm things down so your body understands that it's time to rest. To set the stage for sleep, it is important that we relax and darken the mind.

For example, if you take a hot bath before going to bed, this will create a drop in body temperature, causing your body to begin preparing for sleep. By showering with warm water, your body temperature slows down metabolic functions such as breathing, digestion and heart rate. Your body will understand it's time to slow down and relax. If you have a habit of listening to music before going to bed each night, your body will be conditioned to listening to music at night being the bedtime signal.

It's about habits and conditioning. Take at least half an hour of rest before bedtime to do breathing or relaxation exercises to clear your mind. The purpose of this shutdown time is to tell your brain that it's time to relax, relax and sleep.

## *Sleep in a cool room*

Those who have trouble falling asleep often have a higher core body temperature immediately before falling asleep compared to their healthier counterparts. Therefore, this group of insomniacs needs to wait at least 2 to 4 hours before their body temperature drops and sleep begins.

Research shows that the optimal room temperature for sleeping is between 16 and 20 degrees Celsius. When you're trying to sleep, your brain enjoys the cold environment.

Sleeping in a cold room also helps combat aging. Helps release anti-aging hormones known as melatonin, a potent antioxidant that fights inflammation, strengthens the immune system, prevents cognitive decline and cancer.

There is a saying that those who go to bed early and get up early live longer. It makes a lot of sense considering that sleeping in a cold room reduces neurodegeneration and oxidative stress. I can go on and on about the anti-aging benefits of having a good night's sleep in a cold environment. But the key to increasing the production of anti-aging hormones in your body is to get adequate sleep.

And the first step in doing so is to create an optimal sleeping environment by lowering the bedroom temperature. Lack of sleep has many harmful effects on physical and mental health. Ultimately, it can put your life at risk. So be sure to fix your sleep habits, and you can start doing so by creating an optimal sleeping environment.

## *Pause in the sweat*

Exercise early. It's no secret that exercise improves sleep and overall health. But a study published in the journal Sleep shows that the amount of exercise they do and when they exercise make a difference. The researchers found that women who exercise at moderate intensity for at least 30 minutes each morning, 7 days a week, have fewer sleep problems than women who exercise less or exercise later in the day. Morning exercise seems to positively affect our body rhythms, which in turn improves our quality of sleep.

One of the reasons for this interaction between exercise and sleep may be body temperature. Body temperature increases during exercise and takes up to 6 hours to return to normal. This is because lower body temperatures are associated with better sleep. Therefore, it is important that your body has time to cool down before going to bed.

Sleep is a crucial part of our health and healing. Take it seriously and seek the help of a functional medicine professional if you cannot control your sleep. All of this requires discipline and commitment. Once you restore your biological clock and return to a normal sleep rhythm, you will finally enjoy the benefits of a restful, restful sleep.

## *Lifestyle modification for insomnia*

In the previous chapter, we talked about the two fundamental categories of remedies to overcome insomnia. However, these extrinsic factors could not deal with the root of insomnia. Yes, you may feel better after trying those remedies, but insomnia can only be completely cured if the source of the problem is eliminated. Otherwise, there is a high probability that the insomnia will relapse.

So what's the root of insomnia? For many, the main cause of insomnia is poor lifestyle and sleep habits. Simple lifestyle changes can make a big difference in the quality of your sleep.

Although not all insomnia is caused by stress, it is undeniable that people who experience continuous stress are more susceptible to insomnia. In the case of related stress-insomnia, treating or eliminating the stress will alleviate the insomnia. As mentioned in the previous chapter of this book, stress affects the quality of a person's sleep, which can alter their sleep rhythm. Thus, one will find it difficult to fall asleep at night and stay awake during the day.

It is important to manage all parts of your life in the best possible way to make sure you are in a healthy balance. You need to make sure you're getting enough sleep every day. Sleep plays an important role in your physical health. Insufficient sleep for a short period of time can make you feel more cranky and irritable. Long-term effects can be serious: heart problems, depression, stroke, heart attack, to name a few.

According to sleep experts, several studies have shown that when people get enough sleep, not only will they feel better, but they also increase their chances of living a longer, healthier and more successful life.

To overcome insomnia, you must stay away from nicotine, caffeine, and alcohol. All of this will cause the mind to become naturally restless. Having a constant amount of caffeine will force the mind to be more active than it is.

Most people need the energy to start the day, so they chose the stimulant. Caffeine is one of the most popular stimulant options today to ensure alertness and wakefulness in the morning and throughout the rest of the day. However, they are ignorant of the fact that caffeine is one of the main causes of insomnia. It ruins the natural balance between wakefulness and sleep.

Therefore, insomniacs must stay away from these drinks to have a quality sleep. Skip that coffee break, drink a glass of water instead of coffee, which may be the reason you have trouble falling asleep and staying asleep at night.

Besides that, establishing a sleep schedule for you is one of the best self-help techniques for insomnia. It's an important step in overcoming insomnia forever. It is so important to go to bed at the same time of night and wake up at the same time each morning because the body needs consistency. The body likes routine. He grows up with the habit. With a regular bedtime and wake-up time, your body is more likely to stay on track. If you can, avoid alternating schedules, night parties, night shifts, or other things that may disrupt your sleep schedule.

When you have trouble falling asleep, try drinking a glass of warm milk. It is a traditional remedy for insomnia, and there is evidence that it can help you get better quality sleep. Not only does milk help prevent hunger from disturbing your sleep, but it also contains an amino acid called tryptophan, which is converted in the brain into a "relaxing" chemical known as serotonin. Calcium is very pro-metabolic, reducing stress and decreasing levels of parathyroid hormone, which is known to play a role in insomnia.

Not only that, you can always adjust your own daily schedule to include time for yoga or meditation. There is abundant evidence that yoga and meditation can improve sleep patterns, often dramatically. It is important that you have time to relax. These techniques can be done at home for comfort and privacy. It helps to increase the total flexibility of your body, relaxes your mind and destroys your body. Try to spend at least 30 minutes a day either meditating or doing yoga. Typically, meditation and yoga are best done early in the morning, in a quiet place with exposure to sunlight.

For meditation, all you have to do is sit down and clear your mind. Try to listen to soothing music to help you calm down. The moment you get used to the idea of meditating throughout the day, your mind will be able to relax faster at night and therefore it will be easier for you to fall asleep.

As for yoga, you can go to yoga classes with a group of friends or practice at home for more privacy. It will benefit your sleep in many ways. The practice of certain yoga postures will increase blood circulation to the sleep center in the brain, which has the effect of normalizing the sleep cycle.

Remember, sleep is not a lifestyle choice or luxury; it is natural and necessary. So root out the underlying causes, change your diet, drink a glass of warm milk, set a bedtime, do some yoga, and meditate. Follow the tips above and you will eventually get a quality sleep.

## *Disconnection*



 ➢ ***How to combat insomnia***

Fighting insomnia is an uphill battle. When you're trying to cure insomnia, you're actually trying to keep your mind from being too active at night. There's no reason to be afraid to stay awake for countless nights in a row and wonder if it's all going to end.

Worrying only causes sleepless nights. So stop fighting insomnia in your head! All you need to do is 'Turn off' your monkey brain.

At night, you want your mind to slow down to the point where you can fall asleep quickly. Having an adequate amount of sleep helps you stay fully alert the next day, and ensures a good night's sleep. One of the reasons people struggle to fall asleep is because their monkey brain refuses to shut down. More often than not, they begin to think of useless things that are of no use at all, but only prevent them from falling asleep.

Shutting down requires practice. For many busy adults, the only time they reflect on their lives is at bedtime! It's good to reflect from time to time, but not at bedtime. Often, this is the biggest culprit that keeps you from falling asleep.

So for those who want to reflect on their lives, consider getting up earlier to have time in the morning to do so or even schedule some time at night to do some reflection.

> ***Stimulating Night = Bad Sleep***

Another reason people don't disconnect is that they have many activities at night that are too stimulating, making them stay awake instead of feeling tired. Some even love to drink caffeine at night! No wonder people are struggling to fall asleep! So stay away from coffee, cell phones, laptops, TVs when it's time to go to bed. Avoid activities that force you to think and require physical exertion at night. And most importantly, avoid the 'blue screen' of electronic devices.

> ***Never miss another night's sleep***

Another key to falling asleep is to

program your sleep. Most people don't do that. Instead, they choose to fall asleep only when they are tired. But what they should do instead is establish their routine and schedule their bedtime. In case of repetitions, your mind will be conditioned to turn off when the clock arrives at the usual time to fall asleep.

Having a regular sleep routine is possibly the best technique to ensure better quality sleep. In fact, our bodies thrive on a consistent sleep schedule and regularity. Although there is no one-size-fits-all solution, having a consistent sleep routine will definitely help defeat chronic insomnia once and for all.

# How to 'turn off' at night

The first thing you should do after you've had dinner and cleaned up for the night is turn off any of your electronics. Having your phone or computer on when you are preparing for bed will stimulate your brain and, over time, make it harder to sleep. Admit it, your electronics are addictive and you won't know when to stop.

The light will interfere with your sleep pattern and keep you awake. It is recommended to avoid using gadgets at all costs at least 1 hour before bedtime.

Reading before bed is fine, but not through your electronic devices. Reading a physical book as a hobby before bed actually helps you prepare for sleep. It's better not to read in your room. You are encouraged to read in another room as you do not want your mind to be active in the room in which you need to sleep. Once again, to condition your mind to shut down the moment you enter your bedroom. If you can completely relax while reading a book, then it's okay to do so while lying in bed. Otherwise, it's better to read in another room.

Next thing you can do is listen to music and write any kind of reminder you need for the next day. Music will help calm your mind and eliminate stress. Try to listen to music that is softer and slower in rhythm. Listening to anything that is loud or exciting will stimulate your mind and make it harder for you to fall asleep. For example, you will find yourself in a state of relaxation when you listen to classical music instead of rock.

Another tip is to plan your days ahead before bedtime. Writing reminders for the next day helps clear your mind.

Staying awake in bed while constantly reminding yourself that you need to remember something will keep your mind active. Think of your notebook as a "throw it and forget it" vault. Just grab a piece of paper and scribble a few notes. It will help you calm down and fall asleep faster.

Another thing you can do is drink a relaxation drink like tea just before going to bed. However, be sure to stay away from caffeine, alcohol, and high-sugar drinks. A good cup of tea can calm your mind and help your body relax.

This is also an excellent way to create

time for yourself. A time to rest and relax. You can do this while reading or listening to music. If you don't find pleasure in drinking tea, then consider having a light snack before going to bed. Do not eat anything that is too high in calories and hard to digest. However, a light snack is good because sometimes, the reason you have trouble sleeping is simply because you are hungry.

Another way to ensure a restful sleep is to lower the temperature of your room. The best way to do this is to adjust your room thermostat to be a little colder. Our body is conditioned in such a way that when it enters a cooler environment, it receives a signal that it is time to rest.

Also, why not take a quick shower just before bedtime. Preferably a cold shower to cool down immediately. Otherwise, you can try to get a bed fan, a cooler mattress or take a short walk before going to bed.

All of the above can be part of your bedtime routine. Go ahead, try them out and find out what's best for you and your schedule. In a short time, you will have no problem falling asleep and staying asleep again.

## Conclusion

I hope this book can help and guide you to stop or prevent insomnia. You are free to try any of the tips and strategies listed in this book to ensure a restful sleep. After all, restful sleep is the foundation of your mental and physical well-being. Whether it's artificial or natural remedies, lifestyle changes, or the establishment of a routine, all of this helps prevent insomnia.

> ➢ **So, what to do now? It's time to act today!**

Find out which of these methods works best for you and put them into practice in your daily routine. Write them down and imagine what a normal day looks like when you add these strategies to your routine.

Just by testing them, you can find the best way to overcome insomnia.

Just remember that everything will not happen overnight and that it will take time before you see a change in your life for the better.

Now yes, I wish you the best in your results, and remember, everything is practical; theory without action is of no use to you. It brings everything you learn into real life.

A big hug, your friend, Jorge!

By the way, when you achieve your results little by little, I highly recommend you, if you want to improve your social skills, my book "HOW TO CONTROL SOCIAL ANSIEDAD AND PANIC ATTACKS", is a book that I am sure will help you a lot to avoid any kind of anxiety.  Without further ado, you can find it in the Amazon search engine, like: "How to control social anxiety and panic attacks" or searching for my name "Jorge O. Chiesa"... Once again I wish you success in your results!

www.ingramcontent.com/pod-product-compliance
Lightning Source LLC
Chambersburg PA
CBHW071233240726
48654CB00009B/1036